Dedicated
to
Human Beings
and
Our Maintenance

Paperback ISBN: 979-8-9861693-8-5
E-book ISBN: 979-8-218-43462-5

Exercise.
What?

(Mindful thoughts of a Personal Trainer)

Book 3

Jeff Shammah

Books:

1 Why, 2 How and 3 What:

Should be read in succession and referenced, in order to increase one's use and understanding throughout our lives.

First: Ask for and get help:

Do your research and find a qualified person to guide you on this journey.

Choose: A healthy lifestyle:

That you feel you can practically and realistically execute throughout your life, **instead of instant gratification (Book 2).**

Remember:

The only person that can change a person is **themselves** and once **"you"** make that decision nothing will stop you.

Universal Principle
Book 1

Your first and most important **investment** should be in **yourself,** through a healthy lifestyle.

It does not guarantee immortality, but it will vastly improve the possibility and probability of a **quality** filled existence (life).

We are taught that compounding interest due to early investment will lead to future financial gain.

But, we rarely emphasize that **bad health habits** also compound over time and become increasingly harder to overcome.

Therefore, **Exercise. Why?**

and
now
What?

1. Understand:

that all forms of exercise work **(Book 2)**. Including: cleaning, gardening, caregiving, etc.

2. Accreditation:

teacher needs to have a degree, license, certification or vast experience in the area for which you are seeking help and guidance.

3. Health History Questionnaire/ Waiver:

needs to be filled out and signed in order to provide starting point for exercise program; and for client to accept responsibility for choosing to be involved in exercise program.

4. Distance, timing, speed, weight, repetitions and sets:

are all **individual,** and only **trial and error** will determine what works best for **"you"**. The teacher (trainer) is just a guide to get you started and help along the way.

5. Do not despair or be disappointed that:

there is **not** an exact number or program. Remember that each individual prescription is unique. Your true power and success is found within you, **"not copying"** someone else's routine. Instead, use them as an example and an inspiration to find **"yours"**.

Beginner:
Youth or first time exerciser

Program should include:

Warm-up: "Compound Movements", multiple joint motions that increase the temperature of your muscles and range of motion of joints (lubricate/synovial fluid), in order to prepare them for exercise. This consists of "Full Body" lower and upper body motions that are light and free flowing movements, **not static stretching**. For whatever time is necessary to properly prepare for the activity.

Workout: Should have at least one exercise that addresses all 7 components of physical fitness: muscular strength, muscular endurance, flexibility, balance, coordination, agility and speed. Nothing too hard or challenging, just an introduction (Simple and Basic).

Exercises, weight, sets and repetitions are initially determined by the teacher (trainer). Based on that individual's health history, **not, one size fits all**. Including "Individual Genetic Imbalances" addressed right from the beginning **(Book 2)**, whatever they may be.

Cool-down: Stretching at the end of your program

is the best time for Passive (assisted) or Static (self) stretching. This is when your muscles and joints are at their most fatigued, warm and lubricated (synovial fluid). Therefore most receptive to stretching and increasing one's flexibility. Followed by a basic introduction to meditation (breathing/stillness). This can be done: lying, sitting or standing, all work.

Intermediate

Middle aged or more experienced.

The beginning of a more personal and intuitive approach to your training.

Warm-up: "Compound Movements," your chosen full body and free flowing movements are more prescriptive (personal) in nature. Based on your past experience as a beginner, and learning about what works best for **"you"**.

This applies to any bodyweight movement (calisthenics, walking, yoga, etc.), machine (treadmill, elliptical, rower, etc.), rubber bands, etc., that you may choose.

Less counting (numbers, distance, etc.) and more **"feeling"** for what is necessary to properly prepare on any given day or moment. **Not, a pre-planned program (Book1)**.

Starting to unify the **mind, body and breath** (motion meditation).

Workout: Now, in your application of the 7 components of physical fitness based on your experience gained as a beginner, your workout choices (machines, free weights, swimming, running, etc.) and your exercises (body parts: legs, back, chest, etc.) need to emphasize your imbalances and genetic weaknesses. **Not,** a general "one size fits all program".

The Intensity (how hard or heavy), Duration (how long or number of sets), and Frequency (how often) are also determined by **"your"** personal experience gained as a beginner. **Not**, a pre-planned program.

Cool-down: The modalities now used at the end of your workout (stretching, massage, ice, heat, meditation, etc.) are specific to your individual needs, based again on the experience gained as a beginner. **Do Not, mindlessly repeat your old routines.**

Advanced

Older age or veteran athlete.

Intuitive training (experience), guides your choices (numbers, distance, weight, etc.) during your workout. A now unified: Mind, Body and Breath, provide you with "clarity" and "confidence" (Book 2). Slow and steady truly does "win the race", avoid overtraining.

Warm-up: Gentle, free-flowing, fluid and therapeutic movements (yoga, tai chi, swimming, walking, etc.)

Workout: The continued maintenance of **"Therapeutic"** exercises given to you by your physical therapist, due to genetic deficiencies, illness or past injury is very important. **Do not assume that you are cured.** Prioritize them and add to them, new and more challenging exercises in an efficient manner. Train "Smarter" **not** necessarily "Harder" **(Book 1).** **Emphasize: recuperation, water, nutrition and sleep.**

Cool-down: Leave adequate time after your workout for recuperative modalities: stretching, massage, ice, heat, meditation, etc.

Strength training (muscle) and Cardio (aerobics)

Muscle

Strength training is often incorrectly portrayed as a narcissistic endeavor (ego), examples:

Men: "showing off"

Women: gaining big muscles, "masculinity".

It is neither.

Muscle, whether lean (ballet, marathon runner, etc.) or large (bodybuilder, power lifter, etc.) is the key to locomotion (movement). Transporting yourself from one place to another.

Strength training helps in the slowing down of **Atrophy** (loss of muscle), **Osteoporosis** (bone density loss) and **Metabolism**, by increasing it.

Diet (nutrition) will not and cannot improve these problems alone. In order to maintain **Independence** as we age, in all that life requires of us **(Book 1)**, you must maintain your musculature (muscles).

In order to transport (move) your bones, organs and tissue, maintain and improve your posture and alignment, strength training is necessary.

The heart muscle, brain, along with a strong core (glutes, abdominals and lower back) as well as all the muscles of the lower and upper body, need consistent and continuous exercise. Body weight (calisthenics), free weights, machines, rubber bands, etc., all work in helping to achieve and maintain strong muscles.

Do not rush: it generally takes 8-12 weeks of exercise, 3x per week, **just to begin to form "New Muscle".**

This will require proper caloric intake (calories), from **all three (Book 2):**

1. Carbohydrates (Complex): for energy (fruits, vegetables, whole grains)

2. Fats (Unsaturated): for energy, lubrication of joints and digestion (olive oil, avocado, etc.)

3. Protein (Plant/animal): for repairing and rebuilding of muscle tissue, metabolism, PH and fluid balance, energy (lean meats, poultry, fish and seafood, eggs, dairy, legumes, nuts, etc.) along with adequate amounts of **water** and **sleep.**

Strength training can be done fast, medium or slow depending upon the individuals objectives and goals (power, strength, endurance, speed, etc.), age, health and fitness level.

Progressively, Consistently and **Patiently (Book1)**, and results will follow.

Cardio

The act of strengthening the **Heart Muscle (organ)** and the **Cardiovascular System (blood vessels)** through **Aerobic (oxygen)** exercise.

The heart and cardiovascular system need to be challenged through increased oxygen uptake (breathing). Walking, running, swimming, rowing, cycling, circuit training etc., in order to maintain its strength and elasticity.

This can be done fast, medium or slow. Either low or high impact, depending upon one's objective and goals (marathon runner, sprinter or general health etc.), as well as age, health and fitness level.

Both **strength training** and **cardio** are necessary and need to be treated as part of **one holistic** exercise program. **Not, one over the other.**

Both require adequate caloric intake: complex carbs, unsaturated fats and protein.

Your strength training and cardio programs **should not remain the same as you age:**

Evolution, Progress and **Improvement** require **Change.**

Nutrition
(medicine)

When health is maintained in a **holistic manner** (well rounded), **Exercise, Nutrition** and **Sleep,** there is no need to deprive yourself.

A balanced approach to nutrition which includes: **Carbohydrates** (complex/simple), **Fats** (unsaturated/saturated), **Protein** (plant/animal) and **Water**, leaves room for imperfection. Which is what we are, imperfect beings. **Not deprivation.**

Diet, does not mean less (restriction). It pertains to what you consume (put into your body).

Athletes go on special diets, **often increasing their caloric intake**, in order to perform better.

Bodybuilders in order to increase lean muscle mass and reduce body fat.

The general public in order to improve their health (diabetes, osteoporosis, etc.).

"Skinny" is not necessarily a healthy trait (anorexia/bulimia), it is often a sign of mental health illness.

Please stop depriving yourself, instead improve your relationship with food. Conditioning and unconditioning, based on your past experiences, and improving your understanding of how you got to where you are (therapy).

There are plenty of unhealthy thin individuals, and plenty of healthy heavier individuals.

Food is not the enemy, but the **fuel (sustenance)** to healthier living.

There are many things we still don't understand about why we respond so differently to food, including allergic reactions and intolerances. But, the elimination of food is not the answer.

Nutrition is **Medicine!**

Meditation (self mastery)

What is a Master?

• The understanding of **Oneself**.

The master is the individual in the room who understands how **imperfect they are; and is at peace with that.** Not necessarily right or wrong, just is.

There are two categories and parts to meditation: **Motion** (Kung-Fu, Yoga, etc.) and **Motionless** (standing, sitting or lying down).

Both are practiced around the world in all complete forms of training; and all forms when practiced correctly lead to: **Harmony, Balance** and **Union** of the **One Body (Book 1)**. Through the use of **Breath** and **Postures (breathing exercises)**.

There is no "one right way" to breathe. There are many techniques and methods depending upon the system, goals and health status of the practitioner. Proper guidance from a time tested, experienced and accredited teacher is necessary.

Longevity

While attending a class in college (1982-1986), a professor informed us that a human being had the capacity to live up to 120 years old; and with scientific intervention potentially 140-155 years old.

The question presented to the class was, why were we on average dying so much sooner?

There were many answers: poor air quality, lack of clean water, inadequate nutrition, lack of exercise, stress, etc.

There was no solution given, but the best we could agree upon was possibly **all the above**.

As a personal trainer, I have recounted this lesson to my clients and as you can imagine, often, to eye rolling and disbelief.

Now 40 years later we are being made aware of "Blue Zones" around the world where people regularly live to 100 or more years old, and articles and news reports on centenarians. Science is beginning to take a more serious approach to analyzing these "outliers" (exceptions). We need to study those who take proper care of themselves, **not** just report on those who don't. Otherwise, we become experts on what not to do, instead of what to do.

For the majority of my career as a personal trainer, I have worked with individuals between the ages of 40-90 years old. Several for 30 or more years each. Teaching exercise to them from their 40's into their 70's, and 50 year olds into their 80's. Through marriage, children, divorce, cancer, aids, various illnesses and injury, and even death.

What I have learned from them thus far is that **Longevity** requires:

- **Knowledge** (continued education)
- **Proper nutrition** (food and water)
- **Love** (of self and others)
- **Exercise** (maintenance)
- **Sleep** (recuperation)
- **Income** (money)
- **and Imagination** (will, hope and faith)

In order to translate into **"Quality"**.

Symbols

Book 1: Why?

Recognition and Understanding

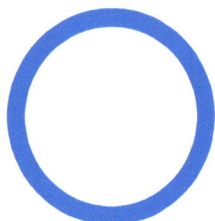 **Everything is "ONE"**

Book 2: How?

Practice

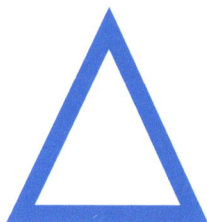 **Balancing and Coalescing**

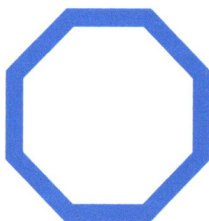 **Leading towards Holisticity**

Book 3: What?

Unity

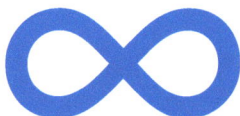 **"ONE" Infinity**

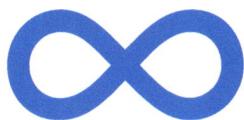

Infinite Possibilities

Facts? I don't necessarily believe in facts. But instead, in our current level of understanding.

What I am most aware of...is how much I don't know (Book 1). There is nothing wrong with saying **"I don't know?"**. Science (life) is a **?**. Searching for and asking questions, not repeating facts.

I often worry that we as humans no longer have or form our own opinions. We seem to be puppeteered or puppets, being given our opinions by others and social media. Rather than listening to all sides and coming to our own individual conclusions.

In order to do this, we need to unplug and reboot ourselves.

As a personal trainer, whenever someone has entrusted me with their most precious possession "their health", I consider it an honor to help them, and I have always done my best.

Acknowledgment

HOPE

To: Yourself **(oneself)**.

We all have a **"Self"** that is at the same time, **Individual** and part of a **Whole**.

We, Us, Our, day to day struggle to be the best that we can be at any given moment or time; for ourselves, our families, our friends and our fellow human beings is why we exercise.

"Life is an Exercise"
Happy Training!

Credits

Photography

Susie Lang

Design

Jeffrey Shammah with Gloria Gregurovich

www.ingramcontent.com/pod-product-compliance
Lightning Source LLC
Chambersburg PA
CBHW040938030426
42335CB00001B/37